D0482648

ESSENTIAL OILS

A LITTLE INTRODUCTION TO THEIR USES AND HEALTH BENEFITS

CERRIDWEN GREENLEAF

ILLUSTRATED BY
ANISA MAKHOUL

RP MINIS

PHILADELPHIA

RP Minis™
Hachette Book Group
1290 Avenue of the Americas, New York, NY 10104
www.runningpress.com
@Running_Press

Printed in China

First Edition: April 2021

Published by RP Minis, an imprint of Perseus Books, LLC, a subsidiary of Hachette Book Group, Inc. The RP Minis name and logo is a trademark of the Hachette Book Group.

The publisher is not responsible for websites (or their content) that are not owned by the publisher.

Library of Congress Control Number: 2020940708

ISBN: 978-0-7624-7265-9

LREX

10 9 8 7 6 5 4 3 2 1

CONTENTS

INTRODUCTION

Essential oils have the power to
heal, to cheer, and to soothe,
as well as to boost your brain
and mood. These ancient oils,
utilized by everyone from
Egyptians to Native Americans,
have been used for thousands
of years, and today are easily
available online and in stores.

This mini guidebook is intended to give you an overview of the top one hundred essential oils from A to Z. Included in the pages that follow are both carrier oils (crucial if you're making a healing potion application for your skin) and essential oils (used to dilute carrier oils while not lessening the power of the essence). We've also included a few fruit essences, which are essential oils that carry the flavor or scent of the fruit.

No matter how delightfully scented, please remember that you should never ingest any of these oils. Instead, use them to create a relaxing home, filled with positive energy; for healing applications; and for all manner of practical magic and spell-work, if that suits you. Our hope is that this mini book will be a handy guide so that when you are experiencing stress, anxiety, and general aches and ailments, or if your mood, mind, and spirit need a lift, you can find the essential oil in these pages that is the perfect match for you. Take good care of yourself; you are very much worth it, and the better you are, the better our world will be.

HOW TO USE
ESSENTIAL OILS

Essential oils are highly con-
centrated extracts of flowers,
herbs, roots, or resin extract,
sometimes diluted in a neu-
tral base oil. Try to make sure
that you are using natural oils,
rather than manufactured,
chemical-filled perfume oils;

the synthetics lack any real energy. While you are learning and studying, find a trusted herbalist or a wise sage at your local metaphysical shop; usually the sage's years of experience offer much in the way of valuable knowledge. Be careful when working with essential oils; use them in conjunction with carrier or base oils so that they do not irritate your skin.

Even diluted, we suggest that you wear clean cotton gloves when preparing oils and do not get the oils in your eyes. You can avoid any mess by using oil droppers.

The best base oils to dilute essential oils are cold-pressed vegetable and seed or nut oils. The most affordable oils are sunflower, safflower, corn, and grapeseed. Add essential oils to your base oil at a ratio of 1 drop per 5 milliliters. Twenty drops of an essential oil amounts to approximately 1 milliliter, so add 20 drops to 100 milliliters of base oil.

Rub one to two drops of oil in cupped palms and take a long, deep breath, or rub one to two drops of oil into your temples or wrists for full body relaxation. A few drops of an essential oil from a dropper in the bath or shower are sufficient for therapeutic use, and a few drops in water in a diffuser will fill a room with healing molecules. A drop on a cotton ball or a cotton pad will also gently diffuse the oil into the air for an instant sense of calm. You can also experiment with mixing and matching oils.

Here's another helpful tip: Try placing a few drops in a small bowl of very hot water. Shut the doors and windows and the essence will permeate a room in five minutes. This is an easy way to create a nice ambience in a room with a soothingly scented air.

Part 1

ESSENTIAL OILS

Essential oils have been used both magically and medicinally for centuries, and are extracted from flowers, grasses, shrubs, herbs, and trees. If you'd like to enhance your immunity and your mood, turn to these scentful oils to alleviate anxiety, respiratory ailments, headaches, and so much more.

Agrimony

Used since ancient times and
very highly regarded as an
all-purpose healer for the body.
Turn to agrimony for help with
sleep; it is a protective herb,
which brings about a sense of
well-being and ease. Remember
to incorporate agrimony essential
oil in your wellness rituals.

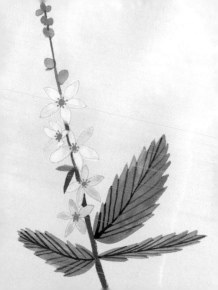

Amber

Derived from the resin of tree sap, amber will ground and balance your personal energy. Amber is also beneficial for purification, psychic shielding, and protection.

Angelica Root

From the beautiful flowering
angelica plant, associated with
the energy of archangels.
This heavenly essential oil has a
fresh and peppery scent,
which promotes peace,
harmony, and good health.

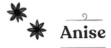

Anise

This essential oil has a wide variety of uses and is excellent for promoting renewed vitality and as a topical in combination with carrier oils for therapeutic massage. Anise carries a strong scent of licorice; makes for deep, peaceful sleep; and protects you from nightmares.

Basil

Effective against depression, worry, and fatigue, basil is used in making perfumes, as well as in aromatherapy. Extracted from the leaves of a basil plant, this oil promotes alertness, lifts your mood, and, as a bonus, repels insects. The scent of this splendid oil is often spicy and warm. A must for money magic.

Bay

This soothing essence is extracted from bay laurel leaves and has magical properties for both physical and mental healing. With an herbaceous scent, bay oil is the perfect choice for relieving migraines and sore muscles, and it's invaluable for psychic development, removing hexes, and attraction magic.

Benzoin

A powerhouse that will connect
you more deeply to your soul
and the realm of spirit, it is also
a great comfort in times of
trouble. In olden times, it was
used to ward off evil spirits and
it is still used for that purpose in
some parts of the world today.
Benzoin oil protects us from the
bad and brings many blessings.

Bergamot

Bergamot's origins can be traced to Southeast Asia, where it was prized for its spicy and floral scent. Bergamot oil is most often used to lift your mood and alleviate stress; it's like liquid sunshine. Send anxiety packing with bergamot essential oil; also exceptional for house magic.

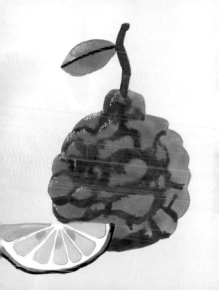

Birch

Utilized by Native Americans
for centuries in cleansing
ritual work and as a medicinal.
Beloved for its sweet, minty
sharpness, birch oil stimulates
and purifies the body and soul.
It is also good for grounding,
and cultivating a practical and
productive mind-set.

Black Pepper

Derived from the common peppercorn, this oil promotes emotional wellness and relaxes the nervous system, Black pepper oil can be administered topically for stimulating the senses and engendering courage. It is also a protectant and can help keep bad energy and bad people out of your home.

Camphor

Extracted from the wood of camphor trees, this oil has many anti-inflammatory and antibacterial properties. It's often used to treat skin irritations, congestion and coughs, and toenail fungus, and it relieves joint pain.

Cannabis Flower

This essential oil has a rich and floral scent, and is widely utilized to create a relaxing atmosphere. It is very calming, helps alleviate insomnia, and will bring pleasant dreams that may also be prophetic. Not to worry: The THC content does not exceed 0.08%.

Caraway

Strengthens mental alertness and enhances memory. Caraway essential oil will protect your aura and conjure up visionary dreams if you sprinkle a couple of drops on your pillowcase at night before sleep.

Cardamom

With a rich and spicy scent, this essential oil is ideal if you're looking to deepen your spirituality through magical workings. It has a strong feminine energy and brings out generosity and openhearted love. If you want to have greater happiness in love, try cardamom in romance rituals.

Carnation

Comes from the sweet small
flower by the same name, and
offers steadiness and strength.
Carnation will uproot buried
emotions and help you process
them, so that you can renew
and reset. It will improve
communication and open
your mind and heart to
new experiences.

If someone close to you has been ill, carnation oil will boost stamina, help release the sadness of sickness, and promote a return to joy.

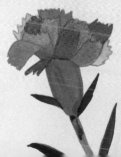

Carrot Seed

A warm and deeply comforting oil that soothes the soul by keeping anxiety and stress at bay. It contains antimicrobial, antioxidant, and anti-inflammatory benefits, making it a great anti-aging agent for the skin. Carrot seed oil enhances empathy, is pleasingly grounding, and removes spiritual blocks.

Cedarwood

Frequently a component of
perfumes, fragrances, and,
ironically, insect repellants.
Cedarwood oil's woodsy aroma
provides a plethora of healing
benefits and is valued for its use
as an anointing oil, as well as for
protective energy in your home.

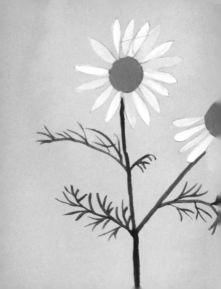

Chamomile

For centuries, chamomile oil
has been used to relieve anxiety,
upset stomach, and indigestion,
and to alleviate troublesome
skin conditions. It promotes
a good night's sleep and
figures prominently in
massage oils, bath oils,
and warm compresses.

Cinnamon

Cinnamon oil stimulates the mind as well as the body. Beloved for its strong, earthy, warm, and spicy scent, cinnamon oil attracts money and blessings, and is excellent for bringing prosperity and protection. It also serves as a great topical oil and contains anti-aging properties by enhancing circulation beneath the skin.

Cistus

Extracted from the flowers of
the rock rose, this essential oil's
aroma mimics that of Sun-ripened
fruit in the summertime: sweet,
fragrant, and with hints of warm
honey. If you feel disconnected
from yourself on a spiritual level,
cistus will restore and rebalance
your soul, and can help you handle
fear, sorrow, and worry.

Citronella

Best known for keeping insects
at bay, citronella oil is a truly
wonderful antidepressant that
is uplifting and encouraging.
The sharp aspect of the scent
clears the mind, too. Using it in
a steam or a diffuser will keep
the energy of your home clean.

Clary Sage

When applied topically, clary sage oil stimulates the skin and circulation while it soothes the mind. It has a distinctly earthy aroma, is a natural antidepressant, and, as the name hints, brings clarity and wisdom. Clary sage also alleviates insomnia, apprehension, and bad dreams.

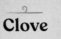

Clove

Derived from clove trees, this strong, spicy essential oil is native to Southeast Asia and is connected to money magic and protection spells. Traditionally, clove oil has been used to fight bacteria and address respiratory conditions, and it's a common pain reliever for toothaches and muscle pains.

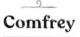

Comfrey

Well-known and widely used by early Greeks and Romans for its inherent curative powers, its very genus name, *symphytum*, from the Greek *symphyo*, means "make grow together," referring to its traditional use in healing fractures. Comfrey, which exudes a strong protective energy, can also keep you from losing both love and money.

Coriander

An essential oil that promotes clear skin, relieves digestive upset, and promotes overall health. With a fresh and fragrant scent, coriander oil aids in relaxation, calms nerves, elevates mood, and is a great aphrodisiac.

Cypress

Originates from the eastern
Mediterranean region; this
mystical oil soothes the soul
and is a balm for those who are
suffering from grief, despair, and
hopelessness. With an evergreen
and lightly spicy aroma, cypress
oil can connect you to loved ones
who have passed away. Cypress
offers strength, energy, and hope.

Dill

Commonly found in Southwest Asia, dill oil gained popularity in the eighteenth century in France when Charlemagne ordered its mass cultivation due to its powerful healing properties. This fresh and bright oil calms the body and quiets nervousness and anxiety.

Eucalyptus

Native to Australia, this fresh and minty oil offers medicinal, antiseptic, and pharmaceutical benefits. Its powerful properties are most often released by placing a few drops of the oil in water. Eucalyptus oil is an all-purpose therapeutic for coughs, colds, and insect bites, and can alleviate respiratory distress.

Fennel Seed

Fennel seed oil has a buoyantly spicy and slightly licorice smell that opens the mind and expands understanding. In a diffuser, this helpmate essential oil works well for space clearing before spells and rituals. Native to southern European lands, fennel seed oil is very stabilizing; it will focus your mind and help in handling difficult work or challenges.

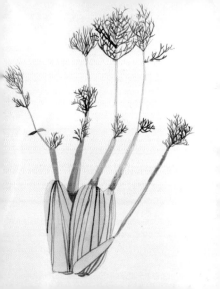

Fenugreek

In use since ancient times, fenugreek oil has a distinctly woodsy and pleasantly pungent scent. It is packed with anti-inflammatory properties that reduce puffiness, inflammation, and acne. It's useful for relieving pain and in cleansing rites.

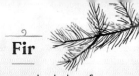

Fir

Also known as the balm of Gilead, this oil comes from the balsam fir tree and has been in use since ancient times. Fir oil is associated with forest spirits and tree magic, and Druids claimed it helped with shape-shifting. It is an awakening essential oil that rebalances heart and mind.

Frankincense

Native to regions of northern Africa, this earthy oil is perfect for clearing blocked nasal passages to promote better breathing. Its benefits can also be obtained by massaging it into your pressure points. An ancient essence that has long been considered precious in the New Testament, frankincense is prized for its use in magical workings.

Geranium

Extracted from the South African *Pelargonium graveolens*, this sweetly floral oil is a true anti-inflammatory that is said to enhance circulation and reduce high blood pressure. Geranium offers emotional stability; releases negativity, stress, and depression; and lifts your mood, as well as boosting your immunity.

Ginger

Ginger is vigorous and revitalizing, and heightens desire and comfort. Native to southern China, ginger essential oil is very much a protector and is believed to ward off ghosts, negative spirits, and harmful energies. It will also spice up your love life and is used for romance rituals. Ginger is a

money attractor and will draw
wealth toward you.

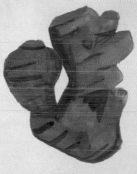

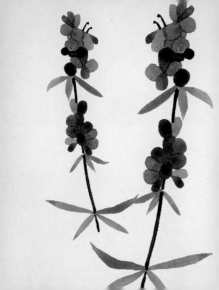

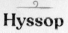

Hyssop

Native to the Mediterranean
region and rich in spiritual
properties. Hyssop oil aids in
the release of grief, sadness,
and depression. This minty-
scented protective oil can be
used for space clearing and
purifying your home.

Jasmine

Derived from the jasmine flower, this mood-boosting, stress-busting essential oil sparks sensuality and inspires feelings of positivity, confidence, and pure bliss. Jasmine oil has been used for hundreds of years, particularly in parts of Asia, to treat depression, anxiety, and insomnia.

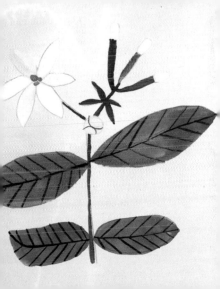

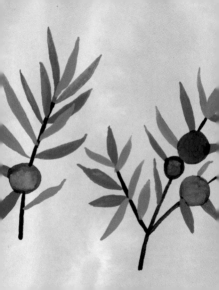

Juniper Berry

Exudes a feminine energy
and is sacred to earth deities.
This essential oil emits a sweet
and woodsy aroma that makes
it a great addition to an
aromatherapy regimen; it
also works as an anointing
application and has strong
space-clearing properties for
use before spellwork.

Lavender

Lavender is soothing, calming, nurturing, and relaxing. This versatile essential oil is a natural antibiotic, antiseptic, sedative, antidepressant, topical treatment for scalds and burns, and a powerful detoxifier. Lavender promotes healing, and the lovely scent has a calming effect that is widely used in aromatherapy.

Lemon Balm

A sweet and lemony essential oil that is ideal for boosting the immune system and calming emotional distress. Because of its herbal undertones, this cold-pressed oil also helps alleviate grief, loss, and sadness; it is truly a balm for many ills.

Lemongrass

Native to Asia, lemongrass has long been used to repel negative spirits seeking to enter the home. The sharp and bright citrus scent of this essential oil can lift up those who are feeling blue or in a rut. Lemongrass is calming and balancing with a protective energy; it can help point you in a direction for a fresh start in life.

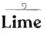

Lime

Comes from the fruit of the
citrus tree. Traditionally, lime
oil's bright and fresh aroma is
great for clearing any blocked
energy channels and releasing
creativity. It is a spirit lifter.

Linden

A lovely oil to have on hand, as it brings love and luck, linden can also create contentment and peace of mind. This essence can overcome sadness and open the heart to new friendships and even new romantic love. Using linden oil in your spells and house magic will make for a happy home.

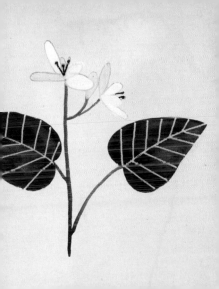

Mandarin

Has been in use since twelfth-century China, where it was beloved for its divine citrus scent and applications as a medicinal for both body and mind. This richly fragrant oil brightens moods and emotions, and alleviates stress and insomnia. Mandarin can help you reconnect with your inner child and the innocence of youth.

Marjoram

Made from a woodsy herb that has a pleasantly fresh smell, marjoram lessens fear, loneliness, and grief. It is very powerful and can even help souls find their way to the beyond. It's helpful for overcoming woe and keeping a happy heart, and is an abundance attractor.

Mimosa

Mimosa has a lightly honeyed scent and will abet self-esteem and self-love. It will help you relax and promote a deep, dream-filled sleep. Try mimosa oil in a steam bath or as a perfume to instill confidence and surround yourself with love.

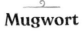

Mugwort

Has long been used in magical
workings, starting in Mesopotamia
and expanding to Europe, Asia,
and now the rest of the world. It
is used by shamans to achieve
heightened levels of awareness.
Mugwort helps alleviate
headaches and soothes
anxiety to restore mental
balance and calm.

Myrrh

A precious essential essence
from prebiblical times, myrrh is
prized for being a warm and lightly
musk-smelling oil. Hailed for its
considerable anti-inflammatory
benefits, myrrh is great for reducing
pain and calming blotchy skin. It's
also an excellent anointing oil for
candles and lamps, and will connect
you to the sacred dimension.

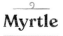

Myrtle

Pressed from the eucalyptus
plant—which was dedicated
to the goddess Aphrodite in
ancient Greece—this slightly
sweet and camphor-scented
oil offers balancing benefits.
It can be used to brighten your
mood, prevent allergies,
and clarify and cleanse
emotional blockages.

Narcissus

Has roots in Greek mythology, and is indeed a visionary essence. Narcissus oil takes you to the realm of imagination. If you want to have intense dreams to feed your creativity, narcissus can bring this to you. Try using it in conjunction with more grounding essential oils such as western red cedar, vetiver, and birch.

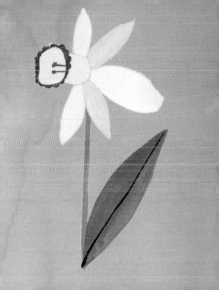

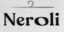

Neroli

Extracted from the bitter
orange tree, originally
cultivated in Egypt, Algeria,
France, and Spain, this essence
contains regenerative qualities,
making it a perfect topical to
alleviate upset skin and even
reduce redness. Neroli is an oil
of the goddesses with a gentle

feminine energy that both lifts emotions and helps overcome fear, worry, anger, and panic.

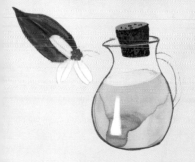

Nutmeg

A warm, spicy essential oil
that is sweet and somewhat
woodsy. Nutmeg blends
beautifully with other essential
oils in the spice family and
strengthens the combination.
Nutmeg is very lucky and is
wonderful in money magic. It is
also fortunate for love and instills
loyalty in a relationship.

Oakmoss

Oakmoss has an earthy energy to match its name; it can ground you and remind you of what you are supposed to accomplish in your life. Oakmoss is very uplifting and brings inspiration. It's an essential oil that is associated with women's wisdom, it is an attractor of abundance, and it's highly recommended for money spells.

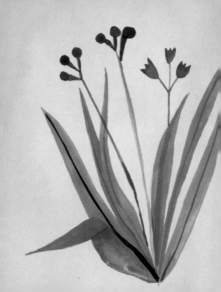

Palmarosa

A sweetly scented essential oil
with a hint of lemon and rose. Also
referred to as the Indian germanium,
this oil contains great benefits
as a topical for skin and is both
smoothing and soothing. It also
mends a broken heart and can
be used in heart-healing spells.
Palmarosa will connect you to a
higher vibration and angelic energy.

Palo Santo

Meaning "holy wood" or "wood of the saints," palo santo is a resinous and richly scented essence that offers benefits of protection and purification and has been used by Native Americans and shamans for millennia. Palo santo is also very good for addressing bad breath, overcoming headaches,

lifting depression, and replacing
negative energy with positive.
It is commonly utilized in
aromatherapy and for
soothing massages.

Patchouli

This aromatic herb is woodsy, sweet, and spicy, and is often used to treat skin conditions and swelling, and to ease colds, headaches, and stomach upset. It's also known for its antibacterial and antifungal properties and is sometimes used as an insecticide.

Peppermint

A wonderful therapeutic for headaches, stress, tension, skin irritations, and depression. It is not surprising that peppermint oil is regarded as one of the world's oldest medicines. It is first rate in money magic and healing work, and can also be useful in divination.

Pine

Renowned for its clean
scent, pine will restore your
spirit when you feel gloomy.
This earthy and fresh-scented
oil is very useful in house magic,
and is associated with longevity
and nature spirits, especially
those of the woodlands
and farmlands.

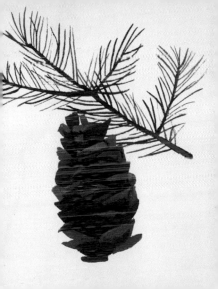

Rose

A favorite because of its perfumed scent, rose oil is distilled from rose petals and used primarily as a fragrance. Originating in the southern Andes, rose oil brings youthfulness, enhances self-esteem, aids circulation, and relieves tension. It's great for nourishing

and hydrating the skin, and
will envelope you in a delightful
and mood-elevating aroma. It's
also very useful in love spells
and in energy management.

Rosemary

A woodsy and sweet-smelling oil that is used as a healer to fight flu, coughs, headaches, depression, muscular stress, arthritis, rheumatism, fatigue, and forgetfulness. You can also put a couple of drops in the bath to make aches, pains, and sniffles go away. It is unusual in that it can both relax you and

stimulate your mind. Rosemary
has a very cleansing energy
and can imbue your home with
coziness and contentment.

Rosewood

Great for easing its user
into a restful night's sleep,
rosewood oil can be used
to calm restlessness and to
overcome the blues. It has very
balancing energy, can alleviate
burnout, and prompts renewal
and a youthful feeling.

Sage

Gaining popularity in the Middle Ages, this spicy and uplifting oil, which has been around for a very long time, contains natural antidepressants, and offers antibacterial and stress-reduction properties. It's great for aromatherapy to reduce your anxiety and clarify your conscience.

Sandalwood

Has been used for centuries
in traditional Chinese medicine
and in East India as a popular
ingredient in Ayurvedic
medicine. Sandalwood has
a woodsy scent and can be
found widely in perfumes and
air fresheners; it is commonly
used in aromatherapy. It is
believed to help treat a number

of ailments, including anxiety, fatigue, indigestion, and insomnia. Sandalwood oil also relieves tension, alleviates dark moods, and causes you to be more alert.

Spikenard

A wonderful, tried-and-true
stress reducer. With an earthy
and woodsy aroma, this oil
is great for calming its user
spiritually and for alleviating
insomnia. Perhaps the finest
quality of spikenard oil is that
it will help you forgive, let go,
and make peace with anyone
who has hurt you, clearing the

way for a fresh start and new beginnings. Turn to spikenard for an emotional reset.

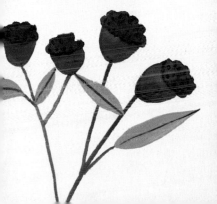

Spruce

Also known as "black spruce," this woodsy oil can promote mental clarity and is grounding when you feel scattered. It was long used as a medicine and in purification rituals by Native Americans, who valued its positive effects on mind, body, and spirit. Smelling the scent in a mist or diffuser can ease breathing, relax you, and help you sleep.

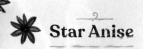

Star Anise

Derived from the commonly
used spice and is prized for its
power to prevent misfortunes
and change your fortune in a
positive direction. Strongly and
pleasantly scented, star anise
essential oil increases psychic
power. It also figures in some
love spells, and can bring
back a lost love.

Tangerine

Has a very bright aroma
that is wonderfully rejuvenating
and stimulates mental clarity.
Tangerine essential oil will bring
a happy heart and a clear mind.
It can also be used to support
the immune system and boost
your mood at the same time.

Tansy

Native to the United States, this sweet-smelling oil is a great agent to fight nerve disorders and destructive emotional impulses. This captivating oil brings deep understanding of life. If you need new beginnings, tansy is ideal.

Tarragon

Tarragon's tangy aroma makes it a great agent to overcome worry, upset, and a negative frame of mind. It is quite good at bringing on a restful night's sleep. This oil is a protectant, offering strength and recovery from deep distress, and can be used to heal from a shock and the resulting trauma.

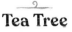

Tea Tree

Used by indigenous Australians for centuries for space clearing and energy management, tea tree oil is a powerful antibacterial, antifungal, and antiseptic with a fresh camphor smell. It can rid your home of negative energy and ward off malevolent spirits. Use tea tree essential oil to clear out and reset vibrations after an illness.

Thyme

An "old-time" curative, highly valued and widely used by the ancient Egyptians, Greeks, and Romans. Thyme confers boldness and is also a restorative to anyone who has faced challenges or experienced great loss. It is a favorite in green witchery and house magic as a protectant.

Tuberose

An intensely rich and sweetly
scented oil that reaches all the
way into the heavens and can
connect you with the spirit realm. It
is transportive and can help banish
low spirits and usher in high spirits.
Tuberose essential oil will reconnect
you to your purpose here on earth
and help you rise above depression,
hardship, and suffering.

Valerian

Initially, this oil came from
Europe and Asia; it engenders
an overall feeling of relaxation.
Valerian can be used to deter
restlessness and promote a full
night's rest. A great and nurturing
aroma for girls and women,
valerian is also an anointing oil,
and is said to bring luck to all
your endeavors. It was

especially popular during medieval times, when it was regarded as a major healing herb for many maladies.

Vanilla

Vanilla oil is obtained from the bean of the same name and has one of the most comforting, heartening, and sweet scents of all. It is excellent in house magic to create a cozy and safe sanctuary, imbuing your home with positive, pleasant energy, and it's useful in spellwork for love and romance. Vanilla raises your personal energy level and helps sharpen mental focus.

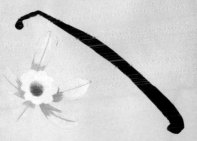

Vetiver

A thick and amber-colored
oil from India, vetiver has been
found to boost immunity and
whole-body wellness. Vetiver
balances emotions and can relieve
nervous tension. Though a very
grounding energy, it can be used
to prevent or reverse curses and
hexes. It is also an abundance
attractor for money magic.

Western Red Cedar

With a woodsy, strong, and refreshing aroma that is powerful for grounding, it is used in nature spells and when working with forest and plant deities. This essential oil promotes longevity and helps you maintain youthful looks and energy. If you want to connect with Mother Earth, use this oil.

Yarrow

Useful for both body and mind, yarrow essential oil has a cooling effect on anxiety, muscle aches, and overall mental wellness. A very pretty plant, yarrow has flowering stalks that were once hung on front doors to ward off evil. This oil brings courage, will make you lucky in love, and can heal a broken heart or spirit.

Ylang Ylang

Ylang ylang's sweet, floral aroma is relaxing and reduces worry and anxiety. This richly perfumed essential oil is a mood-booster, an anti-inflammatory, and an aphrodisiac that benefits both the mind and body. Ylang ylang instills confidence and helps you overcome shyness; it is exceptional in sensual spells and love charms.

Part 2

CARRIER
OILS

A carrier oil is a vegetable oil that is used to dilute essential oils without diminishing the effect of the essence. It ensures that essential oils used topically are comfortable on the skin. Each essential oil carries specific vibrations that hold much curative power. These base oils support other ingredients, including essential oils, and can be a vessel for healing in themselves.

Apricot Kernel

With its warmth and resilience, apricot kernel oil protects and nurtures at every age and stage of life. It works well on both sensitive and mature skin, and is often used in massage oils and bath oils.

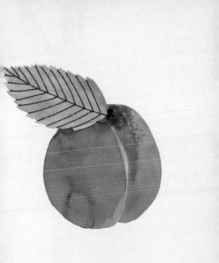

Avocado

This thick, dense, earthy, and nutty oil is a powerful element in any love or money potion. It is nourishing for dry skin and is often used in body creams.

Borage

Borage oil brings a connection
with the higher mind, as well
as courage, a sense of honor,
and the ability to cope with
whatever life sends your way.
It has lots of revitalizing
properties that ease pain in
joints and soothe dry, tired skin.

Coconut

Originating in South and Central America, coconut oil has a plethora of healthy fats that are a great addition to anyone's skin-care regimen and overall health. It also boosts mood and energy. Coconut oil's happy perfume aids memory retention, balances emotions, stimulates weight loss,

and works as a base oil that
supports and blends with
other oils seamlessly.

Evening Primrose

This carrier oil is excellent
for dry, aging skin and can
help treat inflammation and
dandruff. It is commonly
used in soap and
for massage.

Grapeseed

Regarded by some as the "food of the gods" because of how it boosts spiritual growth, grapeseed oil is nourishing for oily skin and popular in skin-care creams and lotions; it's commonly used in massage for its satinlike finish.

Jojoba

Absorbs into the skin
extremely well, bearing anything
it is mixed with. Jojoba comes
from the *Simmondsia chinensis*
plant and is a remarkable
anointing oil. It's an ideal
moisturizer and antibacterial,
and is commonly used to help
deal with depression
and hardship.

Olive

Dubbed "liquid gold" by
the ancient Greek poet Homer,
and rightly so: It promotes vitality,
money, success, and joyfulness.
Its fruity aroma makes it a
natural for homemade soaps
and facial cleansers.

Sesame

Has been used in Ayurvedic medicine for thousands of years, and is rich in omega-6 fats. It absorbs well into the skin, improves circulation, promotes hair growth, and can be used in a nail soak. It's also a stress buster and can help manage mental health.

Sunflower

Permeated with the energy
of our Sun, this oil is powerful
and life-giving, and helps soften
and moisturize irritated skin.
Use it when you desire rapid
growth and amplification
of positive energy.

Sweet Almond

A gentle, all-purpose oil with a strong, nutty aroma. It's a great skin moisturizer that increases the energy of other ingredients.

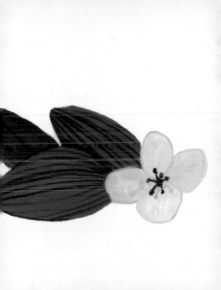

Part 3

FRUIT
ESSENCE
OILS

While we often think of herbs and flowers when we talk about essential oils, it is much less commonly known that fruits may also offer health and healing benefits. While fruit cannot be effectively distilled to create essential oils—they often go through a solvent extraction process instead—their oils can still carry the flavor of the fruit and contain special properties.

Apple

This beloved "one a day" fruit is associated with the goddess Pomona and is suffused with the powers of healing, love, and abundance. This calming and uplifting oil is said to balance emotions and alleviate headaches, depression, stress, and insomnia.

Blackberry

Both the vine and the oil
can be used in prosperity
and money-bringing spells.
Blackberry oil is often used to
help bring relief to irritated,
itchy skin, and its vitamin C can
help fight wrinkles, acne, and
other skin blemishes.

Blueberry

These berries are almost
like an evil eye made of fruit,
as they offer great protection
and can ward off negative
energy and evil. Rich in vitamins
A and B, blueberry oil improves
skin elasticity and offers
relief from itchy skin.

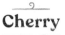

Cherry

Cherries are beloved for their bright red color and taste. Cherry oil is associated with romance, as well as powers of divination, and is used in love spells. This moisturizing oil is found in many salt scrubs and lip balms, and is often incorporated in hair and body treatments.

Fig Seed

Figs hold a special place in
our culture from the biblical
story of Adam and Eve in the
Garden of Eden. Unsurprisingly,
they are associated with sexuality
and fecundity, and are said to
bring luck and safety. Fig tree
oil is rich in nutrients, and
used in cosmetics for its
skin-enhancing benefits.

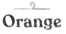

Orange

A light, citrusy oil that restores
balance and lifts moods. A few
drops of this oil will enhance
the potency of any love potion.
Orange sachets and other gifts
with this oil as an ingredient offer
the recipient utter felicity,
making it an ideal gift
for newlyweds.

Peach

Encourages love and enhances greater wisdom. An amulet made with a peach pit dabbed in peach oil can ward off evil. This moisturizing oil is amazing for summer skin, leaving it soft, supple, and with a dewy glow.

Pear

The oil derived from this
uniquely shaped fruit brings
prosperity and a long life.
Somewhat like peaches, the energy
of the pear engenders lust and
love. Pear oil helps to reduce
redness and puffiness,
and promotes
anti-aging.

Pineapple

While renowned as the symbol of hospitality, pineapple represents neighborliness and the energy of abundance. Putting this oil in a sachet and adding it to bathwater will bring great luck. Pineapple oil, which is packed with vitamin C, can help strengthen skin, hair, and nails.

Plum

This rich oil can bring
protection and adds sweetness
to romantic love. It can
help heal dry, cracked skin;
moisturize and add shine to
hair; and is a natural for
fragrances, due to
its fruity aroma.

Pomegranate

This lucky fruit is loaded
with nutrients and its anti-aging
oil promotes cell renewal,
hair growth, and soft,
radiant skin.

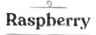

Raspberry

This sweet oil has tremendous
powers for attracting true love
and ensuring safety at home.
It is associated with the Moon
and is sacred to women. Often
found in sunscreens, raspberry
seed oil reduces wrinkles and
dry skin, and promotes
cell renewal.

RECIPES

AND

MORE

Stress-Less Ritual Recipe

This remedy is an excellent way to recharge and refresh after a hectic week. This tincture is most potent right after the Sun sets, by the light of the Moon.

2 drops bergamot oil

2 drops lavender oil

2 drops vanilla oil

1 drop amber oil

4 drops carrier oil

(apricot or jojoba, ideally)

In a small ceramic or glass bowl, gently mix together the essential oils with a small amount of the carrier oil. Gently rub one drop on each pulse point: on both wrists, behind your earlobes, at the base of your neck, and behind your knees. As the oil surrounds you with its warm scent, you will be filled with a quiet strength.

Blissful Balm:
Essential Oils for Love

With this blissful combination of oils, you can summon the spirit of love and harmony any day of the year. Amber, rose, and sandalwood create a sensual scent that lingers on your skin for hours.

25 drops sandalwood oil

6 tablespoons almond oil

5 drops amber oil

3 drops rose oil

2 tablespoons jojoba oil

Mix the oils together in a brown or dark-blue, tightly capped bottle and shake well. You now have an aphrodisiac in a bottle.

Note: Flower- and herb-based aromatherapy essences can also be used in diffusers to infuse the air with the desired fragrance. Many of the most sensual essential oils combine well together: Try a combination of amber and apple, ylang ylang and sandalwood, clary sage and rose, or sweet almond and neroli. If you're using a candle diffuser, rose or orange blossom water is an aromatic and romantic alternative to plain water in the diffuser cup. Other aphrodisiac essential oils include jasmine, patchouli, sandalwood, vanilla, and vetiver.

PERFECT ESSENTIAL OIL PAIRINGS

Use these essential oil combinations to relieve stress, mellow out, and boost your overall mood.

Chill out: Clary sage oil and ylang ylang oil pair up nicely to bring you peace of mind.

Happy hippie: Lavender oil and patchouli oil are a power duo for a quiet mind and upbeat thinking.

Mellow out: Equal parts chamomile oil and rose oil, for a gentle combination.

In your groove: A mix of bergamot oil and basil oil will help you get your groove back.

Sweet serenity: Lemon balm oil and vetiver oil combine for soothing and letting go.

Unwind your mind: Jasmine oil and valerian oil will sweeten up your mood in a jiffy.

MYSTICAL ESSENTIAL OILS

Flowers, herbs, and plants carry potent energy. Use these oils in your spellwork or to help with the following energies.

Astral projection: jasmine, benzoin, cinnamon, sandalwood

Courage: geranium, black pepper, frankincense

Dispelling negative energy and spirits: basil, clove, frankincense, juniper berry, myrrh, pine, peppermint, rosemary, yarrow

Divination: camphor, orange, clove

Enchantment: ginger, tangerine, amber, apple

Healing: bay, cedarwood, cinnamon, coriander, eucalyptus, juniper berry, lime, rose, sandalwood

Joy: lavender, neroli, bergamot, vanilla

Love: apricot, basil, chamomile, clove, coriander, rose, geranium, jasmine, lemon balm, lime, neroli, rosemary, ylang ylang

Luck: orange, nutmeg, rose

Peace: lavender, chamomile

Prosperity: basil, clove, ginger, cinnamon, nutmeg, orange, oakmoss, patchouli, peppermint, pine

Protection: bay, anise, black pepper, cedarwood, clove, cypress, eucalyptus, frankincense, geranium, lime, myrrh, lavender, juniper berry, sandalwood, vetiver

Sexuality: cardamom, lemongrass, amber, rose, clove, olive, patchouli

ASTROLOGICAL ENERGIES FOR EACH SIGN

Use your astrological chart, and the signs of the Sun, the Moon, and stars, to determine which oils are most effective for you. Here is a guide to the astrological associations.

Aries, ruled by Mars: carnation, cedarwood, clove, fennel, juniper berry, peppermint, pine

Taurus, ruled by Venus: apple, oakmoss, rose, thyme, vanilla

Gemini, ruled by Mercury: sweet almond, bergamot, peppermint, clove, dill, lavender, lemongrass

Cancer, ruled by the Moon: eucalyptus, jasmine, lemon balm, rose, myrrh, sandalwood

Leo, ruled by the Sun: cinnamon, nutmeg, orange, rosemary, cypress, lavender, geranium

Virgo, ruled by Mercury: sweet almond, cypress, bergamot, peppermint, oakmoss, thyme, patchouli

Libra, ruled by Venus: marjoram, mugwort, thyme, vanilla

Scorpio, ruled by Pluto: basil, ginger, clary sage, lavender, rose, sandalwood

Sagittarius, ruled by Jupiter: anise, cedarwood, star anise, bergamot, frankincense, lavender, tea tree

Capricorn, ruled by Saturn:
lemon balm, thyme, mimosa,
vetiver

Aquarius, ruled by Uranus:
cypress, lavender, pine, orange,
lemon balm, ylang ylang

Pisces, ruled by Neptune: clove,
neroli, cedarwood, bergamot,
lemon balm, rose

This book has been bound
using handcraft methods and
Smyth-sewn to ensure durability.

Designed by Amanda Richmond.

Illustrated by Amisa Makhoul.

Written by Cerridwen Greenleaf.

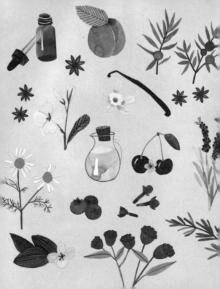